yoga for young people

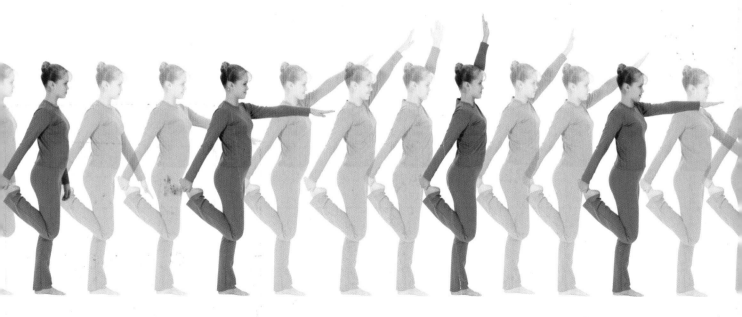

a *flow**motion*™ title

yoga for young people

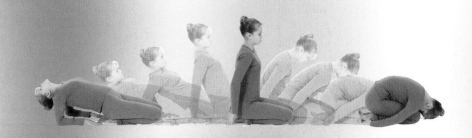

liz lark

Sterling Publishing Co., Inc.
New York

Created and conceived by
Axis Publishing Limited
8c Accommodation Road
London NW11 8ED
www.axispublishing.co.uk

Creative Director: Siân Keogh
Managing Editor: Brian Burns
Design: Axis Design Editions
Project Editor: Madeleine Jennings
Production Manager: Sue Bayliss
Production Controller: Juliet Brown
Photographer: Mike Good

Library of Congress Cataloging-in-Publication Data
Available

10 9 8 7 6 5 4 3 2 1

Published in 2003 by Sterling Publishing Co., Inc.
387 Park Avenue South, New York, NY 10016
Text and images © Axis Publishing Limited 2003
Distributed in Canada by Sterling Publishing
c/o Canadian Manda Group,
One Atlantic Avenue, Suite 105
Toronto, Ontario, Canada, M6K 3E7

ISBN 1–4027–0668–5

Printed by Star Standard (Pte) Limited

a *flowmotion*™ title

yoga for young people

contents

introduction

Whoever is soft and yielding is a disciple of life.

LAO TZE, THE BOOK OF THE WAY, VERSE 76

Yoga comes from India and is a system of study that helps to create harmony. When you practice yoga regularly, you will soon find yourself becoming more aware of everything around you. You begin to notice the tiny details in things, which encourages sensitivity and observation in yourself and in others. These observation skills help you to become a more considerate person, someone who can see clearly and who has a sharp mind.

The word "yoga" means "to link" or "to yolk". Yoga is about connecting all the different parts of the self—the inner and outer, the body, mind, and spirit—in order to maintain good health. To help you understand this, think about the way in which a car needs to be maintained—all its parts need to work well for it to run smoothly. Similarly, an orchestra requires each musical instrument to work in harmony with all the others to perform a great symphony.

There are many aspects to yoga, but the best introduction is through the postures (or asanas, as they are also known) and through the breathing. These are the most accessible, especially for children.

continuing good habits

Although it may seem difficult at first, yoga is actually a natural movement. In fact, it is just like children's play time: absorbing, engaging, relaxing, and replenishing. If you watch young children play, you will see that they naturally lift and arch their spines and work all their muscle groups. Young bodies have not yet been inhibited or restricted by everyday conditioning, so they naturally move much more freely.

If children are encouraged to continue their play time, with a little "yogic guidance," their bodies will retain their natural elasticity and strength as they develop into teenagers and young adults.

Be creative with the postures and always be aware of the center line of your spine.

bodies at rest and in motion

Encouraging children to practice yoga is also a very good antidote to the current television, video, DVD, and computer culture, which stimulates the mind to the detriment of the body. Despite their entertainment value, all of these activities are actually addictive forms of sense deprivation. They fail to encourage one-to-one communication skills and inhibit emotional growth and the development of the essential language skills of listening and speaking.

In previous generations, common teenage leisure pursuits involved going for a walk outdoors in the fresh air, cycling, skating, or running in the park. Today, more and more teenagers spend their free time indoors, sitting down for long periods of time in one position in front of computer screens with headphones on. As a result, a large number

BENEFITS OF YOGA

- develops coordination, balance, and flexibility
- encourages strong bones
- realigns the spine
- tones the muscles
- stimulates blood circulation
- boosts the immune system
- aids food digestion
- helps to eliminate waste products
- massages the internal organs
- regulates breathing
- enhances well-being and vitality
- fosters discipline
- sharpens the mind
- relieves insomnia
- encourages calm feelings
- boosts confidence

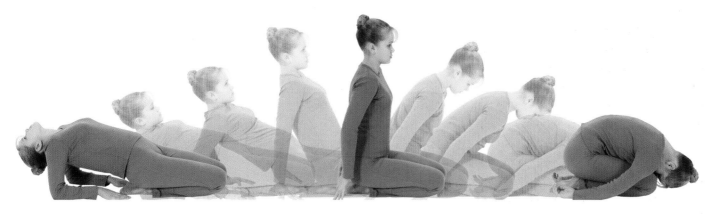

of teenagers suffer from stiff muscles and stooped spines. Tight shoulders and restricted ribcages are also having an adverse effect on breathing and physical self-expression. It's no wonder that in 1995, the German science and nature magazine *GEO* reported that 60 percent of children have poor posture, 35 percent suffer from obesity, 10 percent suffer hearing loss, 38 percent have poor coordination, and more than 50 percent lack the stamina required for running.

eat well, be well

But it is not just sedentary lifestyles and general "couch potato" inactivity that are cause for concern. By the age of 11, it is estimated that one in three children in the UK suffer from obesity. In the United States, reports suggest that obesity among children is vastly on the increase and, it is estimated, will reach epidemic proportions if the situation is left unchecked.

Think of yoga as play that helps connect us to the earth and reach for the sky.

This unhealthy state has come about because a high proportion of a typical child's diet contains processed fast foods that are high in salts, sugars, and unhealthy fats. A poorly balanced diet lacking in wholesome grains and pulses, plenty of colorful fresh fruit and vegetables, oily fish, and natural protein sources, such as meat or beans, is detrimental to good physical health. It will also affect a child's ability to develop mental skills, in particular the ability to concentrate.

Yoga offers a safe, gentle, and highly effective solution to these problems by putting children in touch with their own bodies and helping them to develop a sense of healthy, holistic living. With regular yoga practice, children will very soon start to gravitate naturally toward a more healthy lifestyle and diet.

breathing and concentration

Young children usually find it very difficult to concentrate for long periods because they cannot filter external stimuli. They tend to absorb everything that's going on around them, which can lead to overexcitability and hyperactivity. Yoga helps children to filter out unwanted or distracting stimuli by encouraging them to concentrate on their breath as they practice each posture. Consciously breathing in and out requires a great deal of focus and helps children to concentrate for longer periods and, therefore, helps to discipline the mind.

According to Andrei Van Lysbeth, a Belgian yoga teacher, breathing is our most vital food. Respecting the gift of the breath, treating it like a friend and travelling with it attentively, is essential during yoga. We should breathe through each posture as if fuelling it with energy, which in effect is exactly what we are doing.

You can also kneel and rest the mind for a few moments whenever you need "breathing space."

a considered program

Children learn how to be by observing us. Who we are helps (and may hinder) them become who they are.

RUDOLF STEINER, EDUCATOR

The yoga postures in this book have been specially devised to help children explore yoga in a safe, fun, engaging, and playful way. The program involves stretching and invigorating the body in six ways: bending forward, bending backward, stretching sideways, twisting, balancing, and turning the body upside down. Each of the yoga poses incorporates four important attributes: rhythm, creative flow, grace, and control.

The sequences are easy to learn, flow smoothly from one to the the next, and can be repeated three or more times so they can be memorized. The traditional Sanskrit (ancient Indian) names for each pose have been replaced with animal names and other names drawn from nature.

There are four sections to the program, which progress in a logical sequence that steadily builds skill, focus, agility, and suppleness. Ideally, therefore, the sequences in the book should be followed in the order they are presented, from beginning to end.

The poses in the first section gently limber the body, helping it to warm up from a lying- down position, as if you had just woken up. These stretches make you aware of how the parts of your body connect together.

The second chapter is based on the traditional sun salutation, a way to greet the new day. This sequence of movements brings your attention to the spine, the center line that divides your body into left and right sides like the vertical axis of a tent pole. By developing awareness of the spine early on in life, you will have greater ease of movement throughout life.

The more active and varied sequences in the third section are based on traditional postures that encourage you to stretch sideways, twist, and balance as you complete the program.

The final section focuses on counter-balancing the invigorating postures in the last two sections. To reap the benefits of the entire program, aim to stay in the last, deep-resting posture Savasana for at least five minutes. This helps you to bathe in the benefits of the practice, as if you were drinking a long, quenching drink.

The program should take about 20 to 30 minutes to complete in total, but can be modified according to age. Younger children can do fewer repetitions of each sequence, while older children can do between three and five.

preparing for practice

Whether young, old or very old, anyone can attain power through the practice of yoga.

The Hatha Yoga Pradipika

Unlike many other hobbies, you don't need a lot of expensive equipment to practice yoga. What you will need is some loose, comfortable clothing in which you can move about easily. Natural fibers are preferable to synthetic ones as they absorb sweat and help your body to "breathe."

TIPS FOR RELAXING YOGA

■ Find a clean, clear space that is warm but well ventilated, preferably with fresh air. There should not be any delicate objects or pointy table corners nearby. Make sure the floor is clean and even.

■ Put a yoga mat on the floor and practice on this—it will prevent your feet from slipping, your head from bumping, and your spine from pressing into a bare floor. Always practice on a supporting mat, but make sure it is not too soft; otherwise, you'll bounce or even go to sleep.

■ It's always best to do exercise on an empty stomach, so try to leave one and a half to two hours between eating your last meal and doing the program. You should also wash before and after practice. Since yoga is traditionally regarded as a cleansing exercise, it is good to prepare for the practice by respecting your body and mind. After you have finished drink plenty of fresh water as this will help to flush toxins out of your body.

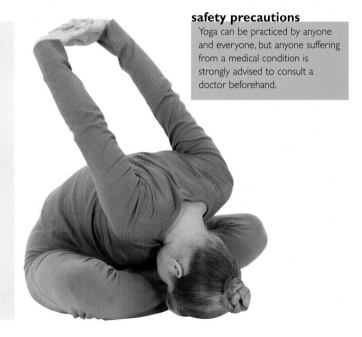

safety precautions

Yoga can be practiced by anyone and everyone, but anyone suffering from a medical condition is strongly advised to consult a doctor beforehand.

resting poses

There are certain postures that help us to relax and feel nurtured and at ease at any time. They can be practiced in any order, at any time, but especially when you feel tired or lethargic.

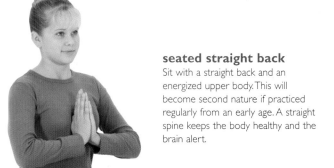

seated straight back
Sit with a straight back and an energized upper body. This will become second nature if practiced regularly from an early age. A straight spine keeps the body healthy and the brain alert.

the corpse pose
(also called savasana)
Lie flat on your back with arms by your side, palms turned toward the sky, and your feet flopping out to the sides. The whole of your skeletal and muscular framework is resting deep into the earth, like a heavy stone.

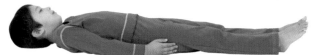

the child's pose
Curl up in a kneeling, torso-folded forward position. This rests the inner body and makes us feel safe and secure from the outside world.

semi-supine resting pose
This is the ideal way to rest your body, relax your spine, and breathe freely.

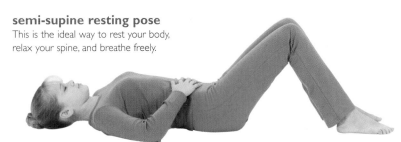

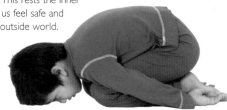

go with the flow

To ensure that children get the very bes out of yoga, the special Flowmotion images used in this book have been created to ensure that you see the whole movement—not just isolated highlights. Each of the image sequences flows across the page from left to right, demonstrating how the exercise progresses and how to get into and make the most of

each position safely and effectively. Each exercise is also fully explained with step-by-step captions. Below this, another layer of information in the timeline breaks the move into its various key stages, with instructions for when you should "exhale" and "inhale," as you move seamlessly from one stage to the next.

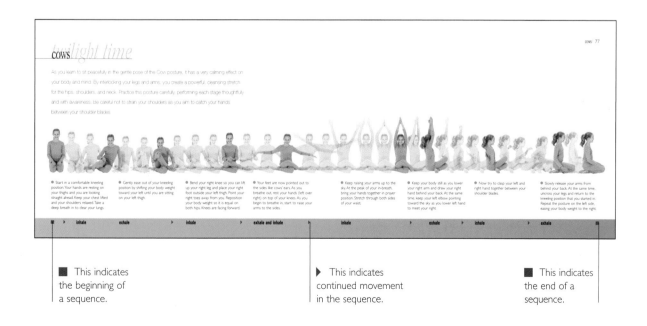

■ This indicates the beginning of a sequence.

▶ This indicates continued movement in the sequence.

■ This indicates the end of a sequence.

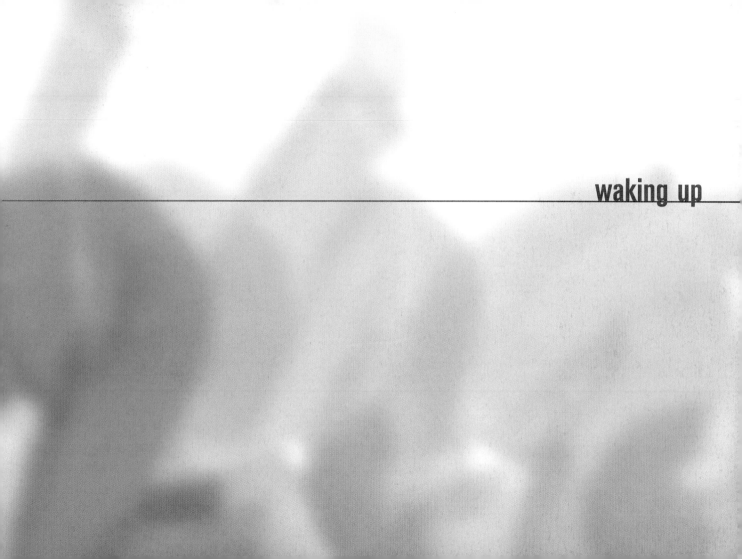

waking up

hedgehog

This gentle limbering sequence begins in the traditional yogic resting posture called Savasana, which means "corpse." It is a bit like playing dead soldiers, where you lie as still as possible. Savasana relaxes your entire body, including your inner organs, and has been practiced by yogis for thousands of years.

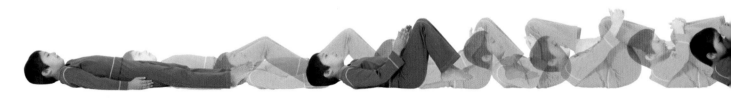

● Lie down flat on your back. Make sure your spine is as straight as a pole and your neck is in line with your spine. Keep your arms relaxed by your sides and let your shoulders drop into the floor like heavy stones.

● Imagine you are floating on water as you stay relaxed. As you begin to breathe in, slowly bend your knees.

● Now, begin to raise your head off the floor as you continue bending your knees up. Bring your hands up toward your shins.

● Lifting your head and knees further toward each other, start to curl up into a tiny ball, the way a hedgehog gets ready to sleep. As you squeeze your knees tight, breathe out.

▶   begin to inhale   ▶   inhale   ▶   exhale   ▶

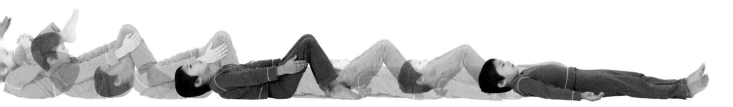

● As you breathe in again, start unfurling as smoothly and as slowly as possible. Avoid any sudden jerks.

● Continue to uncurl like a hedgehog waking from its sleep. As you put the back of your head on the floor, relax your back and shoulders. Your spine should be completely straight.

● Little by little, unclasp your hands from your shins and bring them down to the floor beside you.

● You should now be in the same position that you started from. Take one deep breath in and out, and then repeat the sequence twice more.

inhale ▶ begin to exhale ▶ exhale ▶ inhale and exhale ■

tummy squeeze

This movement massages the lower belly, so it's good to do when you have a tummy ache. It will also help you to digest your food and eliminate it. Always lift your right leg and squeeze the right side of your stomach first, and always breathe out when you squeeze your leg in.

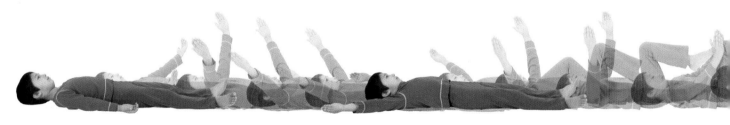

● Begin in the resting or Savasana posture. Lie still and straight as a pole on your back. Let your palms turn upward and your feet flop outward. Take a full breath in and out and then begin to raise your arms.

● Keeping your elbows straight, lift your arms all the way over your head onto the floor behind you. This will help to stretch out your tummy and sides. Keep your head still and the rest of your body relaxed.

● At the peak of the in-breath, the backs of your hands should be touching the floor. Now start to lower your arms back down as you begin to bend your right knee and breathe out.

● Bring your hands around your right knee. At the same time, slowly begin to lift your head off the floor.

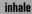 ▶ **inhale and exhale** ▶ **inhale** ▶ **begin to exhale** ▶ **exhale** ▶

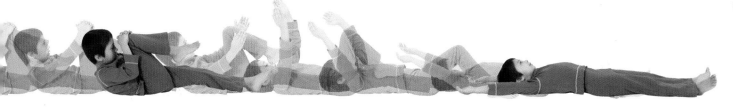

● Now squeeze up tight, like you did in Hedgehog, but this time with only one leg. Aim to touch your forehead to your right knee as if squeezing breath out of your body.

● Undo your hands from around your right knee and take your hands up over your head again.

● At the same time, straighten your right knee and bring it back down to the floor. Your arms and legs are now stretched out fully on the floor.

● Now repeat the movement, doing exactly the same, but lifting the left leg and squeezing the left side of the tummy. If you want, you can do both sides twice more to get a really good tummy massage.

exhale ▶ **begin to inhale** ▶ **inhale** ▶ **exhale**

butterfly wings

This limbering posture is so named because the hips open out like butterfly wings. When your arms are over your head, you make space around your stomach. This helps to relax it so you can digest food and eliminate waste more easily.

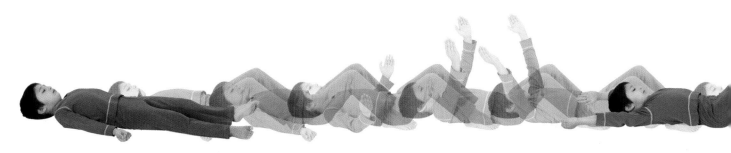

● Start from Savasana, the resting posture. Take a deep breath in and out as you relax your body into the floor. Lie still, with your eyes closed. Imagine you are the caterpillar before it transforms into the beautiful butterfly.

● Start to bend your knees. Slide your feet along the floor so your heels come up toward your hips and your knees point toward the sky.

● Raise your arms up over your head until the backs of your hands are resting on the floor behind you. Keep your hips resting on the floor.

● Let your hips open wide by separating and dropping your knees out to the sides. Your legs are now opening out like butterfly wings.

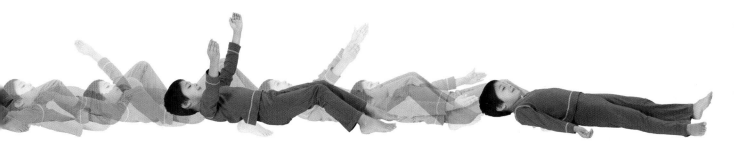

● Now bring your knees together again and rest your feet flat on the floor. Keep your arms outstretched over your head.

● Bring your arms back over your head as if you are drawing an arch in the air. At the same time, straighten your legs back onto the floor.

● While you are doing this, try not to move your body. Keep your shoulders and back relaxed, and make sure they are still touching the floor.

● You are now back where you started, in the Caterpillar position. Take a full breath in and out. Then repeat the whole movement twice more.

inhale ▶ **exhale** ▶ ▶ ■

caterpillar wriggle

Having stretched out your tummy and opened up your hips, you are now going to add a twist. This will massage your back and also strengthen and stretch out the lower back. This movement is good for easing lower back pain.

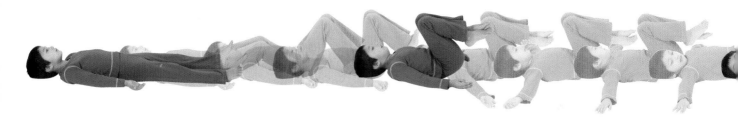

● Start this from the resting posture. Make sure your hands are by your sides, palms facing the sky, and your feet turned outward. Take one full breath in and out as you prepare for the next move.

● Bring your feet together and start to bend your knees so that you can curl your legs up toward your tummy. Keep your head straight and your back still on the floor.

● Begin to slide your arms out to the sides so they are in line with your shoulders. Your body is making a wide T-shape on the floor.

● Turn your hands so that your palms are pressing down into the floor. Tuck your knees up as tight as you can, in toward your chest.

begin to inhale   ▶   **inhale**   ▶

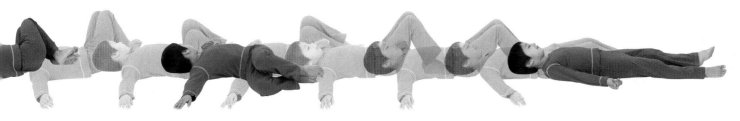

● Lower your tucked-up legs down onto the floor, over to your left side. Your right knee should rest on your left knee. Slowly turn your head to your right side.

● Now slowly turn back to the center so your face and knees are facing toward the sky. Continue turning so you are now facing the left side and your knees have dropped onto the floor over to your right.

● Slowly bring your head and knees back to the center so they are pointing up toward the sky. Keep your hands in the same position so your chest remains open.

● Keeping your head and body straight, slide your hands back down to your sides and straighten your legs. You are now back where you started.

begin to exhale ▶ **exhale** ▶ **inhale** ▶ **exhale** ■

bridge over pond

In our daily lives, we bend forward constantly, so it is important to do the opposite and counter-stretch the spine. It may feel strange, but if you concentrate and do it smoothly and slowly, it is very safe. This posture brings fresh blood into the shoulders, neck, and head, and maintains freedom of movement in the spine.

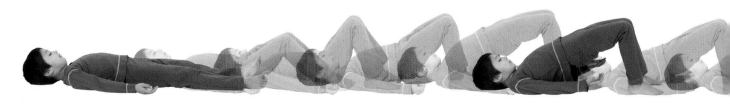

● Start this movement from the Caterpillar Wriggle. Relax your shoulders, neck, and spine as your body sinks into the floor. Take a deep breath in and out.

● Slowly raise your knees so that they point up toward the sky. Keeping the soles flat on the floor, slide your feet in toward your heels so that they are tucked up to your hips.

● Gently, begin to lift your hips off the floor. Avoid sudden, jerky movements. Rest all your body weight on your shoulders. Keep your head still and your neck relaxed.

● With your hips raised, begin to draw your arms together underneath your back. Keep your arms straight as you clasp your hands together.

■ ▶ **begin to inhale** ▶ ▶ **inhale** ▶

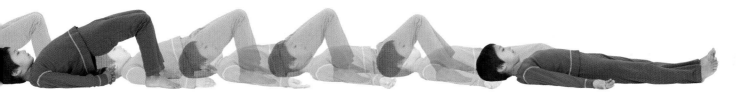

● At the top of your breath, try to lift your hips even higher. Press your arms down into the floor and squeeze the shoulder blades together.

● Now let go of your hands and relax your arms by your side. Keep your head and neck still.

● At the same time, slowly bring your spine down to the floor. Imagine you are a leaf unfurling inch by inch.

● Gently bring your legs down to the floor so you are back in the position you started from. Take another breath in and out and then do the same movement twice more.

end inhale ▶ **begin to exhale** ▶ **exhale** ▶ ■

sleeping mouse

This sequence brings you from a lying down on the floor position to a kneeling curl. It safely massages your spine and lets you rest your head and heart. Try to make the turn as smooth and steady as you can. In traditional yoga, the Sleeping Mouse is called the Child's Pose.

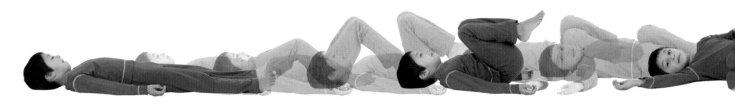

● Start this movement in Savasana. Lie with your back straight, your neck in line with your spine, and your arms by your side. Your palms are facing the sky and your feet are flopping out to the sides.

● Slowly bring your knees together and lift your feet up off the floor. Bend your knees and draw them up to your tummy so the tops of your thighs are touching your stomach.

● With your knees tucked in tight, begin to slide your right arm up past your shoulder.

● Now roll your whole body over so you are resting on your right side. Keep your knees tucked up. Imagine you are waking from a long sleep.

■ ▶ **begin to inhale** ▶ **exhale** ▶ ▶

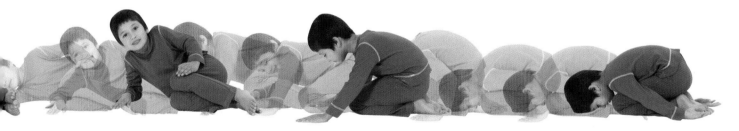

● Continue rolling over to your right side. Then begin to lift your chest up so your weight balances on your right elbow, hip, and thigh.

● Now move into a kneeling position so your body weight has shifted onto your knees. Place your hands on the floor in front of you and look down toward them.

● Curl your tummy and chest over your legs so that your chest is resting toward your knees. Slowly lower your head so that your forehead is resting on the floor.

● At the same time, slide your hands alongside your body until your arms are tucked beside you and your hands are next to your feet. Make sure your palms are face upward. Take a deep breath like a sleeping mouse.

inhale   ▶   **begin to exhale**   ▶   **exhale**   ▶

waking mouse

The traditional purpose of yoga is to become fully awake. This movement is particularly good for awakening the brain and upper body because the raised hips help to flush blood to the upper part of the body. Be careful not to overstretch your neck.

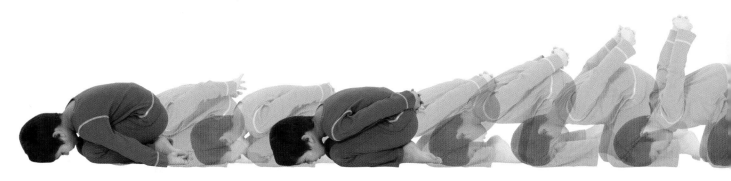

● Before you start to awaken from Curled Mouse, make sure your weight is equal on both sides of your body. Your forehead rests softly on the floor in front of you.

● Lift your arms up off the floor. Then bring your hands together behind your back. Interlock the fingers and rest them on your back.

● Gradually, start to lift your hips up off the floor. Roll forward a little bit so that your weight shifts toward the very top of your head.

● Now raise your arms off your back. Keep your elbows straight and your fingers interlocked.

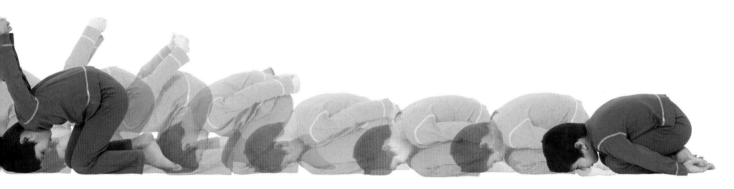

● At the peak of your in-breath, stretch your arms right up toward the sky. Keep your hips high off your heels. You should feel this stretch through your shoulders and neck.

● Throughout the stretch, your feet are in the same position with their tops on the floor and the toes pointing away from you.

● Now lower your hips down onto your heels. At the same time, let go of your hands as you lower your arms down onto the floor so that your hands are beside your heels.

● You are now back in Sleeping Mouse. If you want, you can repeat this sequence twice more to complete the end of the limbering postures.

end inhale ▶ **begin to exhale** ▶ **exhale** ▶ **inhale and exhale** ■

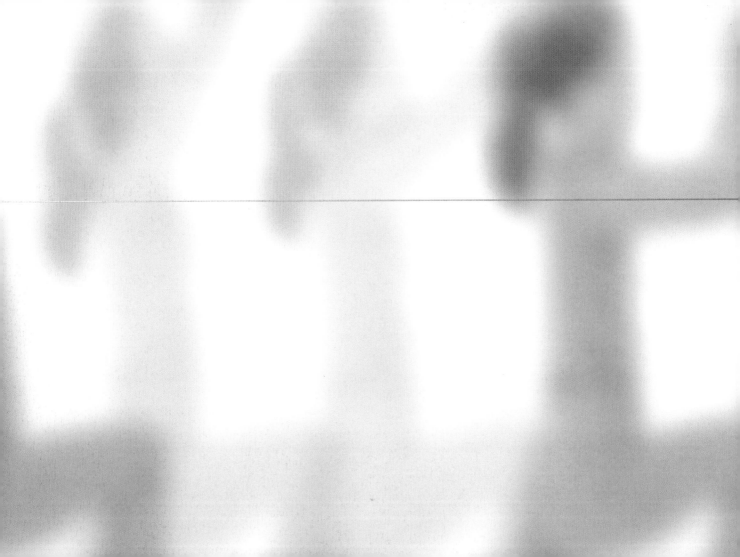

hello to the day

mouse to mountain

From the resting pose of the Mouse, the spine is gently stretched out into a smooth arch—from tail bone, through the neck to the base of the skull. The feet are also stretched as you tuck them into a squat to transform into the tall and steady Mountain pose. In the classical Hatha yoga tradition, the Mountain posture is the foundation standing posture. It is good for encouraging correct alignment and posture.

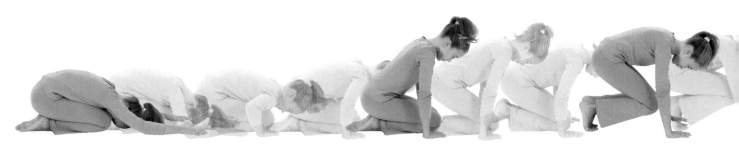

● Start in Mouse position—a resting posture that gently stretches out the back and massages the tummy. Your chest rests on your thighs, toes are pointing away, arms are outstretched, and your shoulders are relaxed.

● Slowly, slide your hands to the outside edges of your knees. Keep your palms flat on the floor and your shoulders relaxed. Gently begin to lift your head up off the floor.

● Keep your chin tucked in slightly toward your chest to relax your neck. Straighten your elbows so your palms are pressing firmly into the floor.

● Now shift your body weight so you are leaning into your hands. Begin to lift your hips up off your heels. Continue to keep your chin tucked in and your toes tucked under.

■ ▶   **begin to inhale**   ▶   **inhale**   ▶   **begin to exhale**   ▶

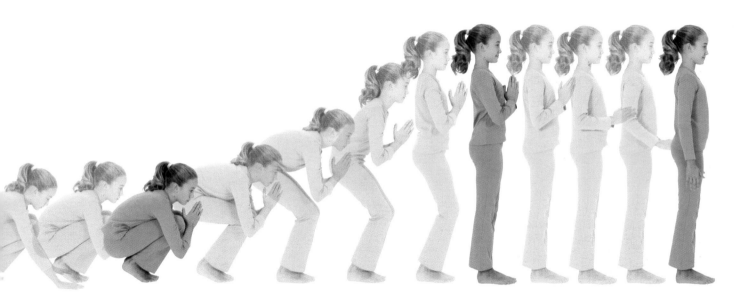

● Shift your weight from your hands to your feet so you are perched on your feet in a squatting position. Lift your hands up off the floor and bring them into Namaste—the universal prayer position.

● Slowly lift your hips up as you breathe in. Press the backs of your heels into the floor as you begin to grow tall. Keep your hands in prayer position and look straight ahead.

● At the peak of your in-breath, stand up firm and tall in Mountain pose. Your spine should be straight as a plant stem and your chest open. Make sure your feet are together and your toes are stretched out like tree roots.

● Imagine the top of your head being pulled up toward the sky as you continue looking straight ahead. Gracefully, lower your arms so they are resting by your sides. Take one full breath in and out in Mountain pose.

exhale ▶ **begin to inhale** ▶ **inhale** ▶ **exhale** ■

reach to the sky

Reaching your arms up over your head will stretch and invigorate your whole body, just like a positive charge. The shoulder roll beforehand helps to loosen and limber your shoulders and open up your chest. When you rise up onto the tips of your toes, try to focus your eyes on a still point in front of you, as this will help you to maintain your balance. If you wobble and fall over, don't worry, just begin again.

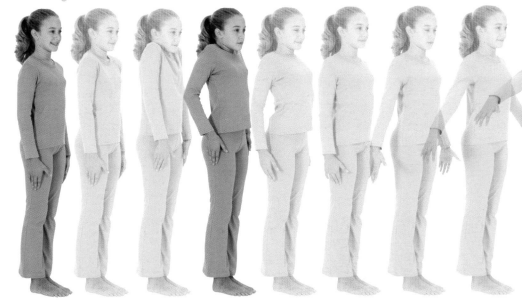

● Standing tall in Mountain pose, take one full breath in and out. As you breathe in, imagine your spine growing up like a plant stem toward the sky. As you breathe out, imagine your feet pressing into the earth like tree roots.

● As you breathe in, roll your shoulders up toward your ears in a big circular movement. As you breathe out, rotate them back and down toward your hips. Keep your hands relaxed by your sides and your legs firm.

● Slowly raise your arms out to the sides. Stretch your hands out, right through to your fingertips. Keep your shoulders relaxed and continue looking straight ahead.

■ ▶ inhale and exhale ▶ inhale and exhale ▶ begin to inhale ▶

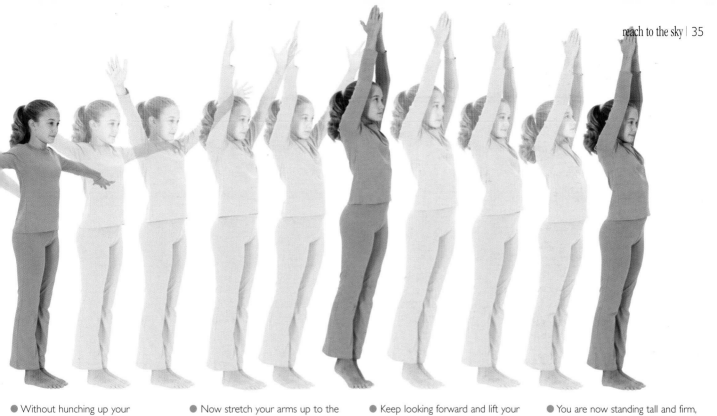

● Without hunching up your shoulders, stretch your hands out to shoulder height, like an airplane's wings. Rotate your palms to face up toward the sky. Keep your feet together and your legs firm.

● Now stretch your arms up to the sky, like the branches of a tree. Bring your palms toward each other and press them firmly together. As you do this, rise up onto the tips of your toes.

● Keep looking forward and lift your chest. As you start breathing out, begin to lower your heels back down to the floor, but try to keep your palms pressed together.

● You are now standing tall and firm, with your arms pointing up like an arrow. Look straight ahead as if looking far out to the horizon. Keep your feet firmly grounded on the floor and take one full breath in and out.

inhale ▶ ▶ **exhale** **inhale and exhale** ■

bow to mountain

This forward bend will massage your tummy and help to relax your neck. It will also stretch your arms and legs and help to encourage graceful movement. The sequence starts from a firm and steady standing position and then moves into a fold, as if diving off a swimming board. Try to keep your back straight all the way through the move. The forward bend gives the brain a refreshing "bath."

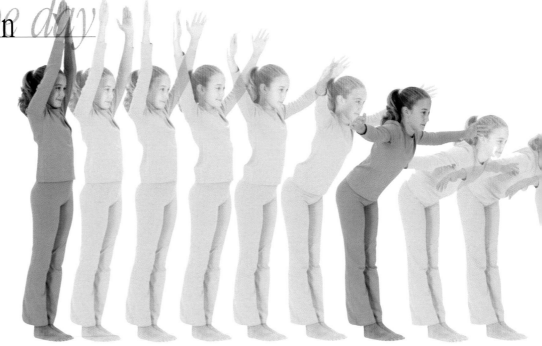

● Stretch your arms up straight like an arrow alongside your ears. Press your palms together. Keep your legs and feet firmly together, and look straight ahead.

● Keep looking straight ahead as you begin to separate your palms away from each other. Your hands remain stretched up to the sky.

● Now start to fold your body, bending from the hips. Begin to open your arms wide out to the side. Keep your chest open.

■ ▶	**begin to inhale** ▶	**inhale** ▶	**begin to exhale** ▶

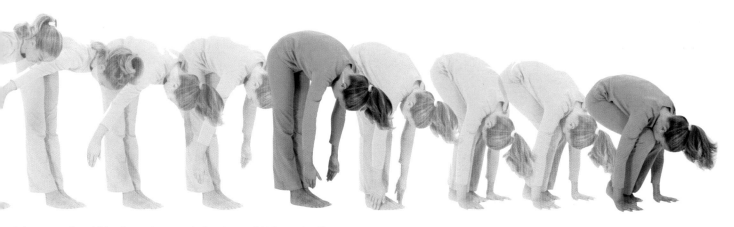

● As you continue folding forward, start to look at the floor. Try to keep your neck relaxed and your shoulders drawn back. Your spine should stay straight throughout the movement.

● Continue to fold forward as if diving in slow motion from the top board at the swimming pool. Drop your arms down beside your legs. Your fingertips should be pointing toward the floor. Your feet should not move.

● Now bend your knees and press your tummy onto your thighs. Place your hands flat on the floor beside your feet. Drop your head so your neck and shoulders are relaxed.

● You are now tucked into a standing forward bend. By bending your knees, you will be stretching your back safely and massaging your thighs.

exhale ▶ **exhale** ▶ **finish exhale** ▪

change to monkey *day*

This sequence involves lunging, so it will give your legs and hips a good, deep stretch. As you reach for the sky, you will also stretch your arms and your heart will be uplifted. The posture starts in a resting forward bend, which acts just like a refreshing bath for your head and brain.

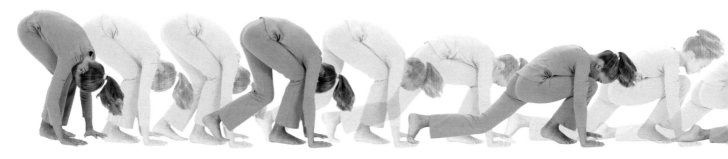

● Start from a resting forward bend. Let your head drop toward the floor so your neck and shoulders are relaxed. Rest your hands lightly on the floor in front of your feet.

● Keeping both knees bent, begin to slide your left foot behind you. Keep your hands on the floor for support. Make sure your head stays loose so your shoulders and neck do not tense up.

● Continue sliding your left leg all the way back until you are in a lunge position and your tummy is pressed into your right thigh. This will stretch out your right hip and help to massage your abdomen.

● Turn your left foot so your toes are pointing away from you and you feel a stretch at the top of your foot. Slowly, begin to lift your chin up.

■ ▶ **inhale** ▶ **exhale** ▶ **exhale** ▶ **begin to inhale** ▶

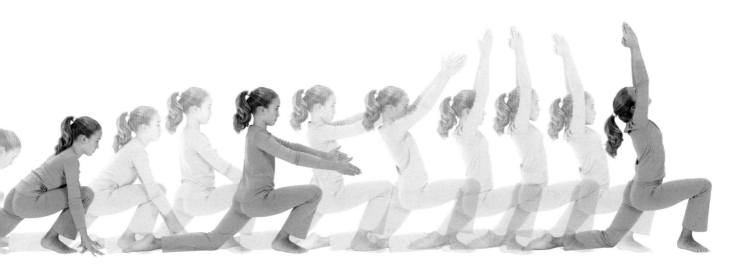

● Stretch out your fingertips and press your hands into the floor to support your chest. Look straight ahead of you and draw your shoulders back.

● Continue lifting your chest as you begin to raise your hands off the floor. Bring the arms forward in a straight line in front of you.

● Imagine drawing an arc with your arms until they are pointing up to the sky. Press your upper arms in toward your ears and continue to look straight ahead as you stretch out the whole of your spine.

● At the peak of your in-breath, look up toward your hands. Continue pressing your palms together, but keep the shoulders relaxed.

inhale　▶　**inhale**　▶　**inhale**　▶　**inhale**

slide to snake

hello to the day

This graceful sequence stretches out your waist and the front of your thighs, and helps you to build strength in your arms and shoulders. As you arch and fold forward, you also awaken your spine. Try to weave in and out of each stage the way a snake does—as fluidly and smoothly as possible. Practicing this sequence regularly will help you to develop your coordination and concentration.

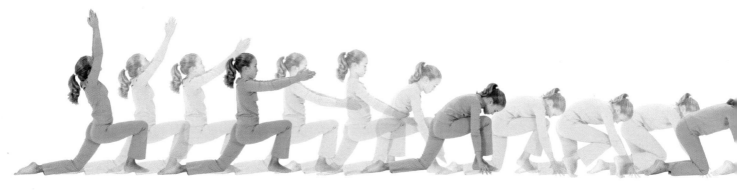

● When you can remain still in your Lunging Monkey posture, take two full breaths in and out. If you can, look up toward your hands, as this will help you stretch open your throat.

● Now slowly lower your arms back down to the ground in front of you. They should be making a smooth arc shape. Look at your hands as you bring them down with control.

● Place your hands on the floor outside your front foot. If you can't place your palms flat, stretch with your fingertips. Keep your back leg stretched out in a lunge so your tummy is pressing on your right thigh.

● Slowly lift up your right foot. Draw it back past your hip so it is lying beside your left foot and you are in a kneeling position. Keep your knees together and your hands still.

■ ▶   exhale   ▶   inhale   ▶

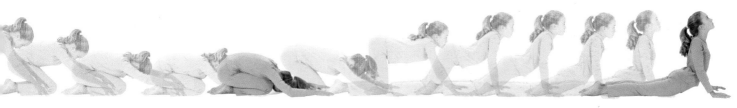

● Keeping your hands where they are on the floor, slowly begin to lower your hips onto your heels. Keep your gaze lowered toward the ground. Lengthen your arms forward and then stretch out your fingertips.

● You are now in Sleeping Mouse position. Breathe in and out three times to relax. Keep your neck loose so your forehead rests on the floor, your tummy rests on your thighs, and your hips rest on your heels.

● As if waking up, start to rise onto your knees and lift up your head so you are looking straight ahead. Dip your spine and gently lower your hips between your hands, like a snake.

● If you can, straighten out your arms and stretch your fingers. Lift your chest and draw your shoulders back. Point your toes away from you. This posture is called the Cobra because it looks like a snake about to strike.

exhale ▶ **inhale and exhale** ▶ **inhale** ▶ **exhale** ■

cat stretch

hello to the day

The cat stretch is the perfect posture for safely awakening and freeing the spine. Watch the way a cat moves so gracefully and effortlessly, and you will soon understand this. Stretching out the spine and opening the chest cavity gives the lungs greater elasticity. Practicing this yoga sequence early in life will help you develop good posture and prevent hunching in later life.

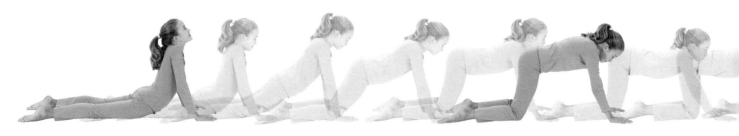

● Start in the Cobra pose with your feet pointing away from you, your chin up, and your elbows straight. Take a deep breath into your heart. This helps to get rid of bad feelings. Imagine you are smiling from armpit to armpit.

● Slowly raise your hips up off the floor, but keep your knees resting there. Make sure your neck is in line with your spine and your chin is tucked in slightly toward your chest.

● Aim to share equal body weight between your hands and knees. Position yourself so your hands are beneath your shoulders and your knees are beneath your hips. Your back is like a table top, parallel to the floor.

● Begin to dip into your Cat arch. Lift your tail bone and your chin up to the sky as you dip your spine into an arch.

■   ▶   **inhale and exhale**   **inhale**   ▶   **exhale**   ▶   **inhale**   ▶

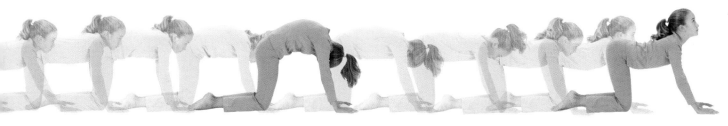

● Now arch your spine the other way as high as you can. Imagine you are pressing the breath out of your body. Curl your tail bone under and tuck your chin into your chest. Do not move your arms and legs.

● When you have breathed out completely, try to arch even higher. Feel your shoulder blades separating away from each other. Try to keep your face relaxed.

● Gently dip your spine again as you begin to repeat your Cat arch. Move through the table-top position so your back is parallel to the floor.

● At the peak of your in-breath, lift your chin and your tail bone up to the sky as you dip your spine again. Keep your arms and legs still as you concentrate on moving only your back. Repeat the stretch twice more.

exhale ▶ **exhale** ▶ **inhale** ▶ **inhale** ■

dip to dog

This movement is just like the way a dog stretches out its haunches. Animals can teach us how to move instinctively again—with ease, grace, and balance. In the Downward Dog stretch, the whole of the back of the body is given a stretch, and the heart and brain are rested and replenished.

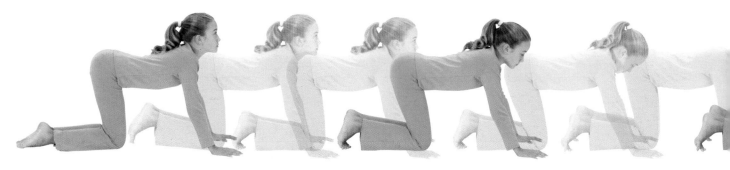

● From the Cat stretch, start to lower your head and gaze. Check that your hands are positioned shoulder-width apart. Press your palms firmly into the floor and stretch out your fingertips like starfish.

● Lift your feet so you can tuck your toes underneath. Spread out your toes and stretch the balls of your feet. Keep your arms straight.

● Take one full breath in and out as you prepare for your Downward Dog stretch. The knees and feet should be hip-width apart. Look toward the floor as you breathe out.

● Drop your head completely to the floor. Remember to keep your neck and shoulders relaxed. Try to keep your back straight so it is parallel to the floor, like a table top.

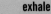 ▶ **exhale** ▶ **exhale** ▶ **inhale and exhale** ▶ **exhale** ▶

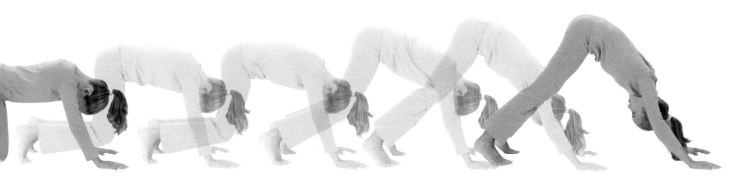

● Press your weight into the palms of your hands and the balls of your feet as you prepare to push your hips up high into the sky.

● Look toward your belly button as you continue keeping your neck and shoulders relaxed. Now, begin to straighten your legs as you shift your weight from your hands to your feet, raising your hips smoothly.

● You should be able to feel a good stretch through the hamstrings (the backs of your thighs) and the calf muscles. Keep your fingers stretched out like starfish, gripping the floor firmly, to stop your hands sliding.

● Draw your chest toward your toes. Aim to stretch your arms and spine in one long diagonal line to the floor. Your whole body is now making an inverted V-shape, with your hips pressing upward to the sky.

exhale ▶ ▶ ▶ **end exhale** ■

return to monkey day

Having stretched both sides of the body in Downward Dog, this sequence complements the first Monkey pose by lunging forward with your left hip to stretch the right side of your body.

By repeating this move on both sides, we learn how to link postures together, as if choreographing a dance. This helps to develop mind and body coordination, especially when the movements are linked with the breath.

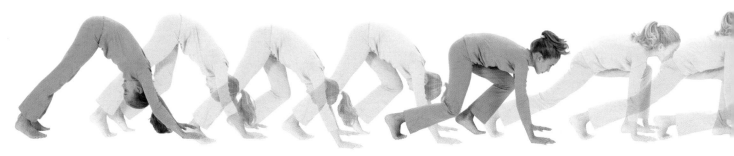

● Start from the Downward Dog position. Your head is drooping toward the floor and you are looking toward your belly button. Your hands and feet are firmly on the floor and your fingers and toes are outstretched. Knees and elbows are straight.

● Begin to lean your body weight into your hands. Keeping your head lowered, start to bend your left knee as you lift up your left foot.

● Raise your head and look forward as you bring your left foot up toward your hands. Keep your left knee bent as you tuck it up by your chest.

● Aim to place your left foot between your hands. Keep looking straight ahead. Your right heel should be rising up high as you stretch the ball of your right foot.

■ ▶   **inhale and exhale**   **begin to inhale**   ▶   ▶   ▶

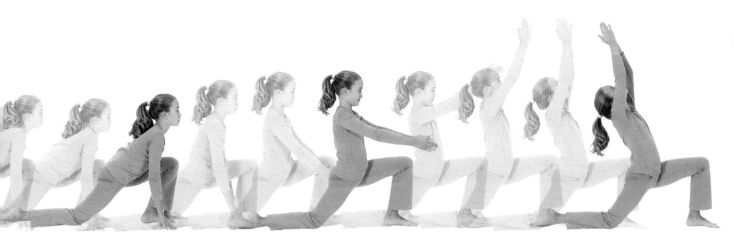

● Now drop your right knee onto the floor as you lunge forward into your left leg. You should feel a good stretch in the front of your right thigh. Keep your shoulders down and your chest open.

● Rest the top of your right foot flat on the floor. Lift up your chest so your spine is straight and your back is vertical. Release your hands from the floor and start to raise them up in front of you.

● Keep your elbows straight as you press your palms firmly together. Try to keep your left knee bent at a right angle so your left thigh is parallel to the floor. Draw your arms forward and up in an arc.

● At the peak of your breath, look up and back toward your hands. Draw your elbows toward each other. Aim to keep your hips in line (both facing forward), and keep your shoulders and face relaxed.

continue to inhale   ▶   ▶   **inhale**   ▶   ■

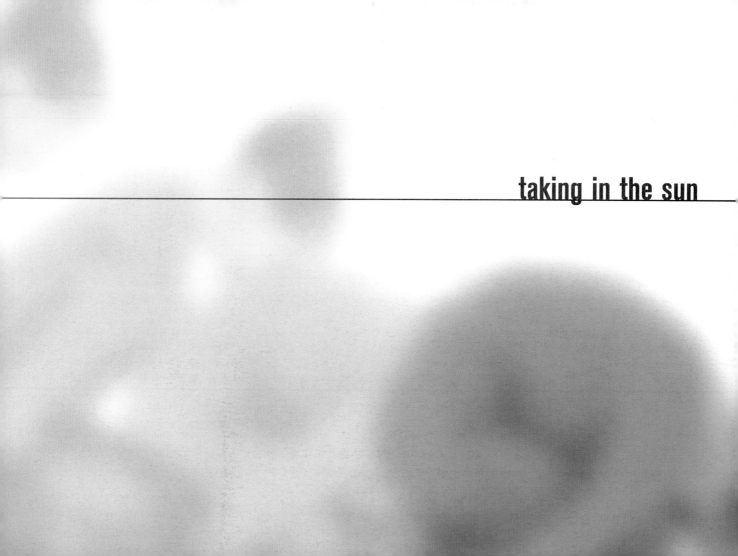

taking in the sun

frog hopping

This movement mimics a jumping frog, hence the name. It is good for developing upper body strength and the squatting position stretches out the lower back and hips.

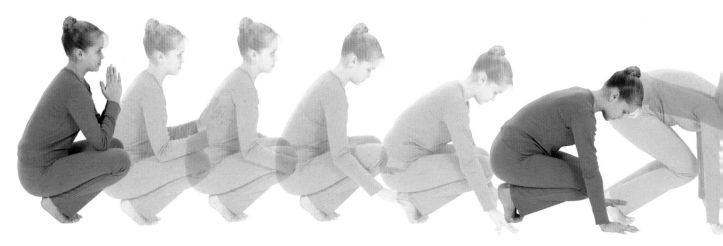

● Perch on the balls of your feet. Keep your knees together and your chest lifted. Make sure to stretch out all of your toes. Place your hands in prayer position and rest your elbows on your thighs.

● Start to lower your hands on the floor. Try to keep your balance and the rest of your body still. Slowly look down toward the floor.

● Place your fingertips on the floor just in front of you. Gently, begin to lean forward so that you start to transfer your body weight into your hands.

● Press your palms firmly into the floor. Having the correct hand position is very important because you will be supporting your whole body weight on your arms as you jump up.

begin to exhale ▶ exhale

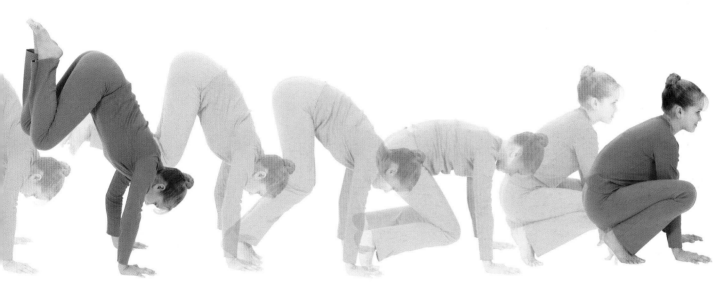

● Now, get ready for your spring. As you breathe in, lift your hips as high as you can as you leap up into the air. Keep your knees bent and tucked in toward your body.

● Keep looking at the floor between your hands. Concentrating on a still point (or gaze point) will help you to maintain your balance. In traditional yoga, your gaze point is called Dristi. This helps to focus your attention.

● As you breathe out, return to your squatting position as buoyantly as possible. Imagine you are a frog landing lightly on a lily pad.

● Lower your hips back down to the heels. This time, make sure your knees are outside your arms, which are held straight. This will stretch your hips and thighs and prepare you for the next posture.

inhale ▶ **exhale** ▶ ■

crow balance

The squat position creates the transition from frog to crow. The crow balance strengthens your upper body and teaches you how to balance with poise and grace. The posture also gives a wonderful hip stretch and develops strong arms. You must concentrate hard to keep your balance, and this training will strengthen your body and help you to focus on other aspects of your life.

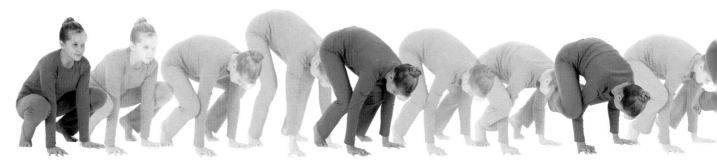

● Perch comfortably on the balls of your feet. Secure your balance by leaning into your palms. Keep your elbows straight and your arms energized. Lean forward slightly and lift your chest. Look straight ahead.

● Lift your hips up toward the sky and look down between your hands. Your knees should be resting on the outside of your upper arms. Continue to lift your hips as you prepare for your arm balance.

● Lean forward as you begin to bring your shoulders over your hands, bending your elbows slightly. Feel the weight shift from feet to hands. Continue looking down to the ground.

● Bend your elbows out to the sides to create ledges with your upper arms. This creates a platform to balance on. Lower your shin bones onto the tops of your arms.

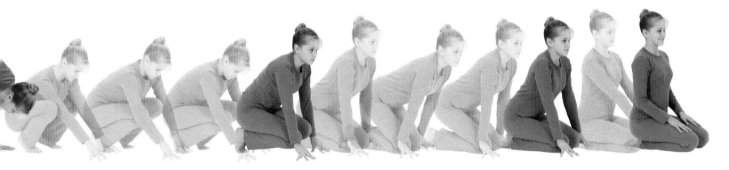

● Lean forward with confidence and when you are ready, lift your feet off the floor. You are effectively crouching over your hands with your feet off the ground, tucked up behind you. Aim to touch your toes together.

● After a few seconds, gently lower your feet back down to the floor as you breathe out. Continue to lean forward as you lower your knees on the floor in front of you.

● Lift your hips slightly so you can flip your feet and point your toes away from you. As you begin to breathe out, sit back on your heels in a kneeling position.

● Bring your spine into a straight line, vertical to the floor. Place your hands on your thighs. Relax your face, neck, and shoulders as you take one deep breath in and out.

inhale ▶ **exhale** ▶ **inhale and exhale** ▶

lion roars

This wonderfully expressive movement helps to stretch out all the muscles in your face, including the eyes, jaws, and tongue. As well as roaring like a lion, you also stretch out your fingertips like a lion's claws. This pose helps get rid of bad breath and cleanses the tongue and throat, thereby enhancing your pronunciation.

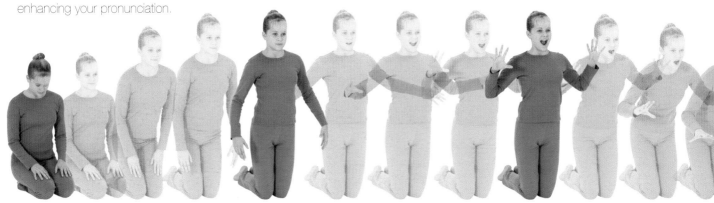

● From your kneeling position, rest your hands gently on your thighs. Make sure your spine is straight and your toes are pointing away from you. Tuck your chin gently down toward your chest.

● Begin to lift your hips off your heels so that you are drawing your body up into a raised kneeling position. Keep your feet and knees together.

● At the same time, begin to lift your hands off your thighs. Bend your elbows as you raise your arms out to the sides. Keep your shoulders relaxed and keep looking straight ahead.

● At the peak of your in-breath, open your mouth out wide as you summon up all of your energy and prepare to...

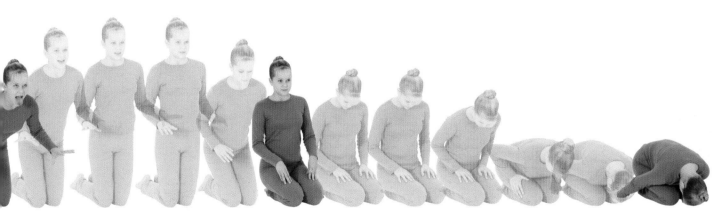

● ...roar! As you breathe out, lean forward. Stretch out your tongue and fingers and roll your eyes to look up. Stretch out your fingers like claws, too.

● Draw your body back up into a straight line, keeping your knees in the same position. Having rid yourself of any negative feelings and tension, take a deep breath and imagine a cleansing wave washing through your body.

● Sit back down onto your heels. Bring your hands back onto your thighs and tuck your chin in toward your chest again.

● As you continue to breathe out, fold your body down over your thighs. Rest your chest on your thighs, with your arms straight alongside your body. Relax your shoulders and let your forehead drop to the floor.

exhale ▶ inhale ▶ exhale ▶ ■

thunderbolt *in the sun*

This movement stretches out the whole of the front of your body as you move into a kneeling backbend. If this strains your knees in any way, just sit with your legs stretched out in front of you. Both sides of the body are stretched evenly at the same time, which can be a real challenge. This posture helps you to digest food and cleanse the abdomen and gives the spine a wonderful arch.

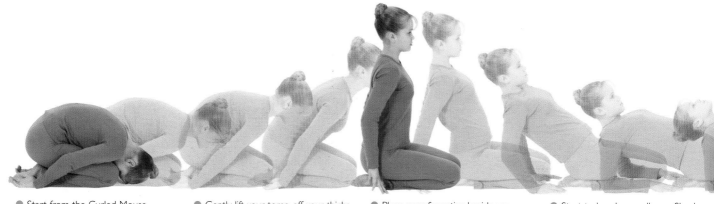

● Start from the Curled Mouse position. Make sure your forehead and shoulders have dropped toward the floor. Close your eyes and take a deep breath in and out to prepare.

● Gently lift your torso off your thighs so you bring your back into an upright position. You should be kneeling comfortably with a straight spine.

● Place your fingertips beside you you. Keep your shoulders drawn back and your chest lifted. Now place your hands flat on the floor a little behind you, with your fingertips pointing inward.

● Start to bend your elbows. Slowly and gently, lean back until your elbows are on the floor and your forearms are lowered behind you.

■ ▶ **inhale** ▶ **begin to exhale** ▶ ▶

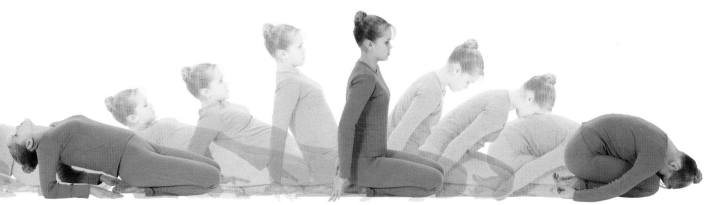

● Keep your chest open and lifted so your heart is raised. As you finish breathing out, gently let your head drop back to stretch and energize your throat.

● Begin to lift your head, tucking your chin into your chest. This will protect your neck as you come back up into a kneeling position.

● Bring your hands up alongside your body. Let your fingertips touch the floor and keep your arms straight. As you begin to breathe out, slowly start to fold forward again.

● Your chest is resting on your thighs and you are now back in the Curled Sleeping Mouse position. If you can, repeat the back bend twice more.

finish exhale ▶ **inhale** ▶ **begin to exhale** ▶ **exhale** ■

eagle
taking in the sun

This beautiful posture encourages strong legs by stretching all the muscles in your limbs. It also helps to strengthen your torso. To master the Eagle pose (the king of the birds), you need to develop a lot of concentration, balance, and determination.

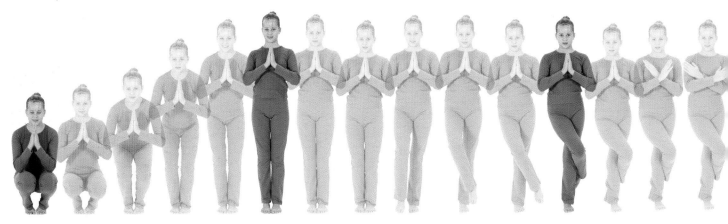

● Start from a balancing squat position. Take one deep breath in and out. This will prepare your rise and transformation into the powerful and majestic eagle.

● Begin to raise your hips up as smoothly as possible. Keep your head and chest lifted and look straight ahead. Continue rising until you have come into a full Mountain pose, with your feet firmly rooted to the ground.

● Keeping your hands in prayer position, bend your knees. Carefully balance on your left leg as you slowly wrap your right leg around your left shin. Hook the right foot around the left calf muscle, if possible.

● Release your hands from prayer position and begin to lower them like wings, right arm over left arm. Keep your spine straight and continue looking straight ahead.

■ ▶ **inhale** ▶ **exhale** ▶ **inhale** ▶

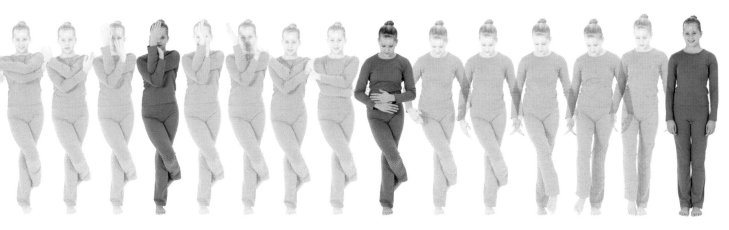

● Maintain your leg posture as you begin to wrap your arms tightly around each other, interweaving your forearms. Try to press your palms together and lift your chest. Keep your hips and shoulders level on both sides.

● Once you have held the posture steady, begin to separate your hands. Keep your shoulders relaxed and stand steady.

● As you continue balancing on your left leg, slowly bring your hands down to your sides. Keep your chest lifted and your shoulders relaxed and drawn back.

● Now, release your legs and bring your right foot back down beside your left foot. Stand tall in Mountain pose and take one full breath in and out. Now repeat the Eagle pose on the left side, lifting your left leg.

exhale ▶ **inhale** ▶ **begin to exhale** ▶ **exhale** ◼

dancer's pose

taking in the sun

The balance required for the Dancer's Pose encourages concentration and coordination. To help keep your weight on one foot, find a fixed point in front of you and focus on it, imagining that you are taking root through your standing foot.

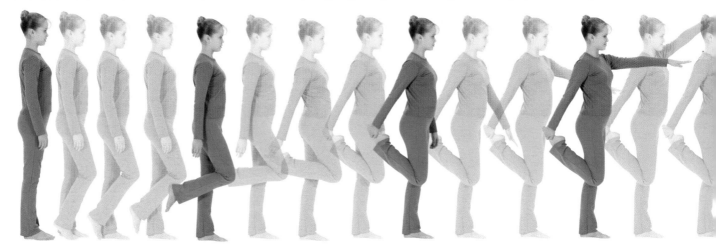

● Stand tall and firm in the upright position of Mountain Pose. Your shoulders are in line with your hips, your hands are by your side, and your feet are together. Look straight ahead at a fixed point.

● Aim to keep your hips level with each other as you slowly raise your right foot behind you. Catch the right foot with the right hand.

● Lift your chest and continue looking straight ahead. Try to keep your knees, hips, and shoulders in equal balance.

● Raise your left arm up in front of you. Stretch out your hand so your arm makes a smooth, straight line parallel to the floor. Make sure your knees are together and your face and neck are relaxed.

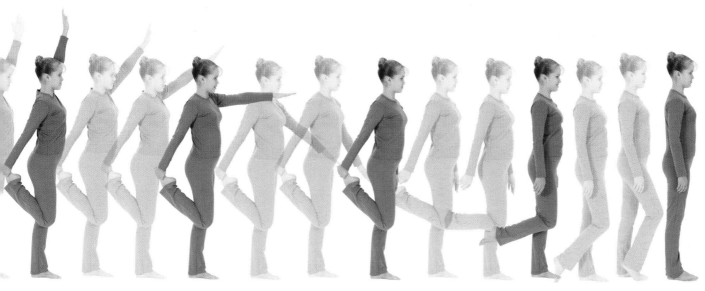

● Continue to raise your left arm up until it aligns with your spine and your fingertips are pointing toward the sky. Enjoy the stretch through the whole left side of your body.

● As you start to breathe out, lower your arm again, as if drawing a semicircle through the air. Stay firm and grounded in your standing leg. Keep looking straight ahead.

● Let go of your right foot and begin to lower the leg down to the floor as your bring your hand back down to your side. At the end of your out-breath, you will be standing once more in Mountain Pose.

● You are now standing firm and upright, with equal weight on both feet. Lift your chest, relax your shoulders, and take one deep breath in and out. Now repeat the sequence again, lifting up your left foot.

▶   **begin to exhale**   ▶   **exhale**   ▶   ■

fairy wings *in the sun*

This powerful arm posture exercises the joints and muscles in your shoulders, arms, wrists, and hands. Putting your hands in the backward prayer position requried to gain such an intense stretch looks just like a pair of fairy wings. The openess this creates in the chest encourages free breathing and helps to get rid of anxiety so you can breathe freely.

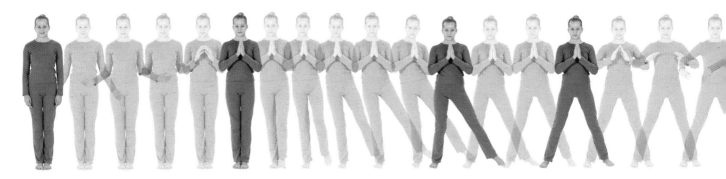

● Begin by standing tall and firm in Mountain Pose. Imagine a sky hook is attached to the crown of your head and is lifting you up so your spine is lengthening out of your pelvis.

● Slowly bring your hands out and up to your chest. Bend your elbows, placing your hands in prayer position.

● Keeping your hands in this position, lift up your left foot and step it out to the side. Your feet should be about 3ft (1m) apart.

● With your feet parallel to each other, slowly release your hands from prayer position. Stretch your arms out to shoulder height and keep your back straight. Your body is now stretched out like a five-point star.

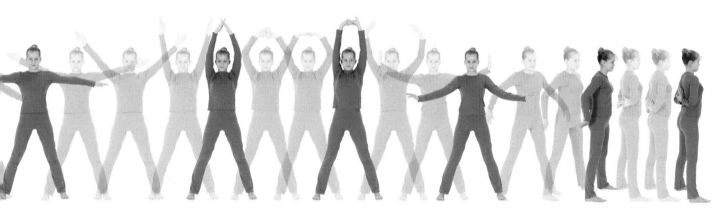

● Now raise your arms up to the sky. Lift your chest up and stretch your abdomen and spine. At the peak of your in-breath, interlock your fingers as you prepare to put your fairy wings in place behind you.

● With your fingers interlocked, turn your palms to face the sky. Stretch powerfully through your arms. At the same time, keep your feet flat and firmly grounded into the floor.

● As you breathe out, slowly release your hands and draw your arms out to the sides. Keep your face relaxed. Lift your chest and broaden your collarbone.

● Bend your elbows and bring your hands behind your back. Press your palms together so they are in prayer position behind your back, between your shoulder blades.

inhale ▶ ▶ **exhale** ▶ ■

fairy folds forward

The position of the arms in this movement helps you to open up your chest and increase your lung capacity. This encourages deep breathing, which keeps the mind calm. Bending forward also helps to bring fresh energy into the top half of your body and soothes the brain and heart.

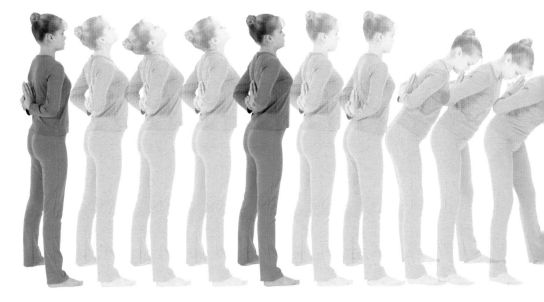

● Keep your arms firmly in place as you tighten your thigh muscles, grounding your feet firmly into the earth. Take a deep breath in and out as you prepare for the next move

● Draw back your shoulders as you begin to lift your head. Look up as you gently tilt your head back and take a deeper breath into the heart.

● Keep your shoulders back and collarbones broad. Begin to fold forward from the hips. Keep your back straight, if possible, and bend your knees a little if your back is straining.

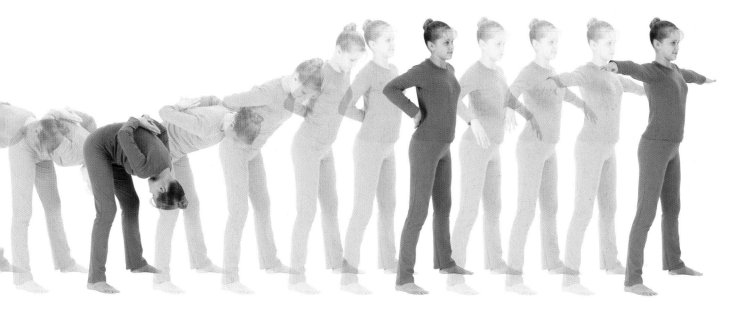

● Aim to keep your elbows (Fairy Wings) in place behind you. Press your palms together, as this will help to keep your hands from slipping down your back. Drop your head so you are looking though your legs.

● Remember to bend your knees a little so you don't strain your back. Keep your feet in place as you raise your body up and return to a full standing position. Lift your chest and keep your shoulders drawn back.

● Start separating your hands. As you breathe out, take your hands out to the side and roll your shoulders back.

● With your hands outstretched to shoulder height, your body is forming a wide T-shape. You are now ready to stretch into starfish.

▶   **inhale**   ▶   **exhale**   ▶

starfish

This posture is good for developing your balance. It may be familiar to you as a "jumping jack," but there is no jumping. Although yoga is a physical activity, it is also about controlling your energy. Being still and moving with awareness requires concentration and focus.

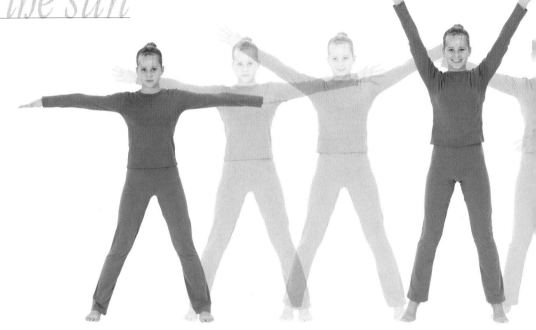

● Start as you have finished Fairy Folds Forward. Your feet are parallel to each other and your weight is evenly balanced. Your arms are stretched out straight at shoulder level. Look directly in front of you.

● Keeping your weight evenly balanced, slowly begin to raise your arms up and out to the sides. At the same time, rise up onto your tiptoes. Reach up to the sky, creating a deep stretch throughout your body.

● Once you feel your spine lengthening, slowly start to breathe out. Gently lower yourself back onto the soles of your feet. Bring your arms back down to shoulder height.

■   ▶   **inhale**   ▶   **begin to exhale**   ▶

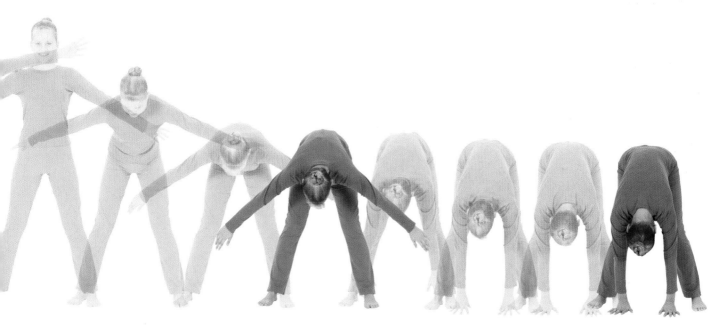

● Begin to bend forward from the hips as you continue breathing out. Try to keep your legs straight and firm and continue to stretch your arms out to the sides.

● Gently lower your head so you can look down at the ground. Continue bending from the hips and keep your arms outstretched, making a semicircular shape as you lower them toward the floor.

● As you ffinish breathing out, place both hands on the floor just in front of you, between your feet. If you can't reach far enough to place your palms flat on the floor, stretch out your fingertips instead.

● Relax your neck so that you can drop your head right down. Take one full breath in and out and feel your spine releasing tension as you relax into the forward bend.

windmill twist

This movement involves turning the spine like a windmill from a standing forward bend. Twisting like this will strengthen and rejuvenate your back. Twists are said to wring out the spine like a wet cloth. Think of your spine—from your lower back to the base of your skull—as a fresh plant stem that you fill with energy. This sequence also helps to develop coordination.

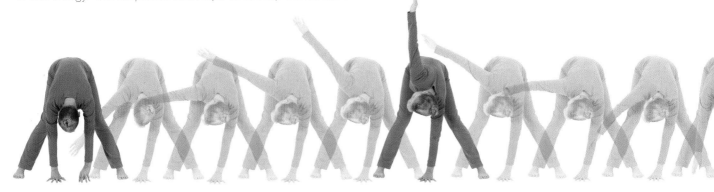

● From the finishing Starfish posture, take one full breath in and out. This will help to relax your upper body over your thighs. If your lower back feels strained at all, bend your knees.

● Place your left hand between both feet so it forms the third point of an equilateral triangle with your feet. Now slowly and smoothly raise your right arm out to the side, so it is turning like a windmill.

● Keep both arms outstretched and your left hand steady on the floor until your right hand is pointing up toward the sky. Turn you face to look at your hand as you raise it. Take three breaths in this full-twist position.

● Now, lower your right arm again. Keep your eyes on your hand as you move it down to the ground.

■   ▶   **inhale**   ▶   **exhale and inhale**   ▶   **exhale**   ▶

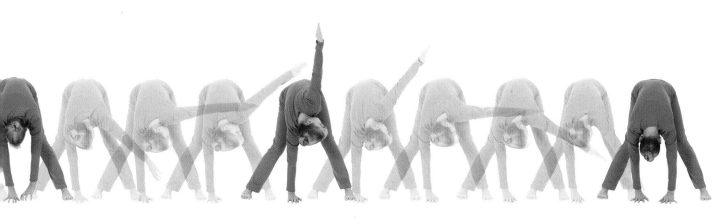

● Place your right hand firmly on the floor in place of your left hand to form the three points of a triangle with your feet. Now, start to repeat the twist on your left side.

● Draw back your left shoulder and keep your chest open as you raise your left arm up to the sky. Look at your left hand, following its arc with your gaze. This helps you to develop your concentration.

● Take three full breaths as your arm reaches to the sky. Slowly lower your left arm to the ground, making a smooth arc in the air. Place your left hand on the floor next to your right hand.

● You have now returned to the starting position of the standing forward bend. Take a deep breath and slowly stand upright. This completes the end of the standing postures.

begin to inhale ▶ **inhale** ▶ **exhale, inhale, exhale** ▶ ■

twilight time

mouse to crocodile

The Mouse Posture in this sequence stretches and awakens your spine in a forward bend, and the Crocodile Posture stretches your spine in an arch. It is important that backbends arch your whole spine, and the Crocodile Posture will open up your upper back, lower back, and also your heart. It helps, too, to massage the stomach. The Cat is the link between the two postures.

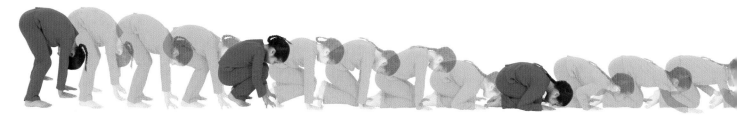

● Begin by standing forward with your hands planted firmly in front of your feet, which are wide apart and parallel to each other. Your head drops down toward the floor.

● Gradually bend your knees, dropping your hips down toward the floor in a squatting position. Lift your hands so only your fingertips are touching the floor. Keep your head lowered and look to the ground.

● Lean your body weight forward into your hands and gently drop your knees onto the floor in front of you. Now, as you finish breathing out, point your toes away from you, kneel down, and curl up into Sleeping Mouse.

● Slowly lift your head and hips up off the floor as you begin to move from Waking Mouse into Crocodile. Slide your hands forward and position them beneath your shoulders.

■　▶　**inhale**　　　**begin to exhale**　▶　**exhale**　▶　**inhale**　▶

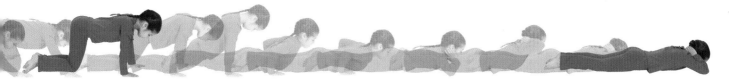

● You are now in Cat posture. Take one full breath in and out, making sure your back is parallel to the floor, like a table top. Your arms and thighs should be vertical to the floor.

● Gently drop your hips between your hands. Start to bend your elbows so your upper body is lying on the floor. Empty your lungs completely.

● Slowly lift your hands off the floor and interlock them behind the back of your neck. Make sure your elbows are pointing out to the sides. Now, gently lift your chest up off the floor, like a Crocodile.

● Having lifted and opened your chest like a yawning crocodile, gently lie back down on the floor, face downward and your hands still behind your neck. Rest and breathe.

exhale and inhale   ▶   **exhale**   ▶   **inhale**   ▶   **exhale**   ■

locust to mouse

The locust posture is good for stretching out and strengthening your lower (lumbar) back and complements the Crocodile stretch, which concentrates on the upper back. By balancing on your tummy, you massage your abdomen and receive a wonderful stretch throughout the whole of the front of your body. This posture lets you feel as if you are skydiving.

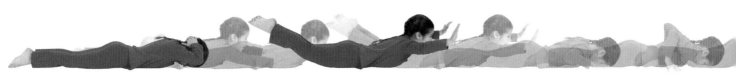

● Begin by resting in Sleeping Crocodile, lying face down. Take one full breath in and out as you prepare to transform into the Locust position.

● Release your hands from behind your head and straighten your arms out in front of you. At the same time, stretch out your legs behind you.

● Point your toes away behind you and stretch out your hands. Arch your body like a bow. Aim to look forward.

● Bring your head back down to the floor, placing your forehead gently on the ground. Relax your legs onto the floor again. Bend the elbows and put your hands beside your ribcage.

■ ▶   **begin to inhale**   ▶   **inhale**   ▶   **exhale**   ▶

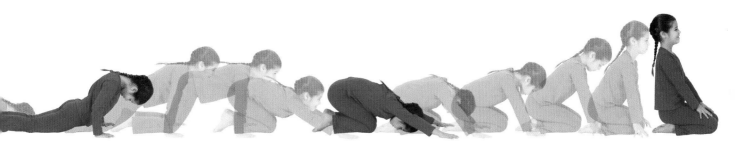

● Now press your palms firmly into the floor. As you breathe in, lift your chest up into a Cobra arch. Follow through by lifting your hips up. Then, place your knees on the floor and your hands beneath your shoulders.

● Move through the Cobra arch, bringing your hips back and lowering them onto your heels. Don't move your hands so your arms lengthen. Drop your head onto the floor. Rest your abdomen on your thighs

● From Stretching Mouse, begin to lift your torso off your thighs in a smooth movement. Keep your neck in line with your spine as you move your hips to your heel so you are now in a seated position.

● Straighten your spines like a plant stem and lift the top of your head up to the sky. Kneeling comfortably, rest your hands on your thighs. Finish by taking a full breath in and out.

inhale ▶ **exhale** ▶ **inhale and exhale** ▶

COWS

As you learn to sit peacefully in the gentle pose of the Cow posture, it has a very calming effect on your body and mind. By interlocking your legs and arms, you create a powerful, cleansing stretch for the hips, shoulders, and neck. Practice this posture carefully, performing each stage thoughtfully and with awareness. Be careful not to strain your shoulders as you aim to catch your hands between your shoulder blades.

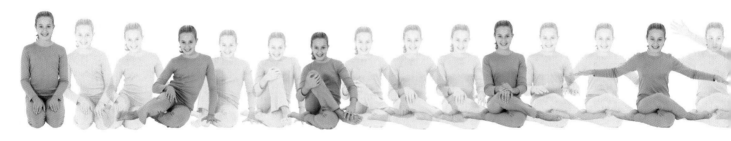

● Start in a comfortable kneeling position. Your hands are resting on your thighs and you are looking straight ahead. Keep your chest lifted and your shoulders relaxed. Take a deep breath in to clear your lungs.

● Gently ease out of your kneeling position by shifting your body weight toward your left until you are sitting on your left thigh.

● Bend your right knee so you can lift up your right leg and place your right foot outside your left thigh. Point your right toes away from you. Reposition your body weight so it is equal on both hips. Knees are facing forward.

● Your feet are now pointed out to the sides like cows' ears. As you breathe out, rest your hands (left over right) on top of your knees. As you begin to breathe in, start to raise your arms to the sides.

  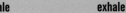 ▶ **inhale**   **exhale**   ▶   **inhale**   ▶   **exhale and inhale**   ▶

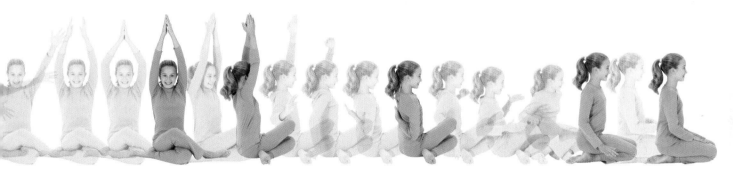

● Keep raising your arms up to the sky. At the peak of your in-breath, bring your hands together in prayer position. Stretch through both sides of your waist.

● Keep your body still as you lower your right arm and draw your right hand behind your back. At the same time, keep your left elbow pointing toward the sky as you lower left hand to meet your right.

● Now try to clasp your left and right hand together between your shoulder blades.

● Slowly release your arms from behind your back. At the same time, uncross your legs and return to the kneeling position that you started in. Repeat the posture on the left side, easing your body weight to the right.

inhale ▶ **exhale** ▶ **inhale** ▶ **exhale** ■

gate for cow *twilight time*

This raised kneeling position involves a side stretch that tones the waist. We have stretched the spine in forward and backward bends, and the Gate for Cow complements this by allowing a deep sideward stretch. In yoga there are six main body directions in which to stretch: forward, backward, side angle (this pose), twist, balances, and inversions. An integrated yoga program will include all of these.

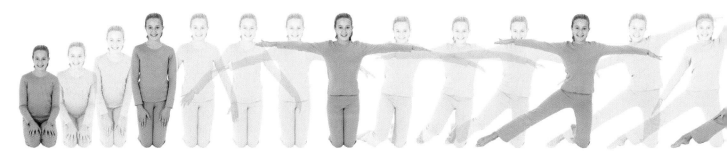

● From a kneeling position with hands rested on your thighs, slowly start to raise your hips off your heels. Continue to look forward and keep your face relaxed by smiling gently.

● Begin to raise your arms out to the sides as if you are blowing up a big balloon. At the peak of your in-breath, stretch your arms out to the sides like airplane wings.

● Gently, slide your right leg out to the side. Stretch it as straight as you can. Plant your right foot on the floor like an anchor to give you stability.

● Begin to raise your left arm up toward the sky and drop your right shoulder down. Place your right hand on your right knee.

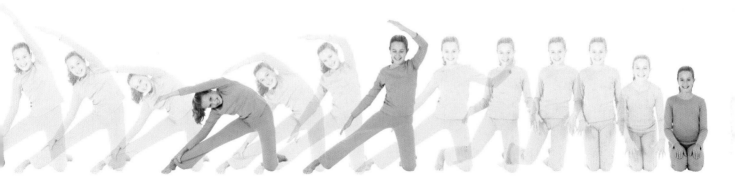

● Stretching both arms, begin to arch your left arm over your head toward your right side.

● At the same time, lean your torso over your right leg as you slide your right hand down your right leg as far as it will go. Take one full breath in and out in this powerful side stretch.

● As you begin to breathe in, draw your torso back up so your spine is straight again. Lift the crown of your head up toward the sky.

● Bring your arms back down to your sides and slide your right foot back so your knees and feet are together. Lower your hips onto your heels, raise your hips and repeat the stretch on the left side with your left leg outstretched.

▶ **exhale**   **inhale and exhale**   ▶ **inhale**   ▶ **exhale**   ■

flower bud closing

In this series of movements, the body is tightly closed up, like a flowerbud that contains all its goodness within. Hugging the body tightly like this helps to massage, protect, and nurture your tummy and heart. It will also give your back a good stretch.

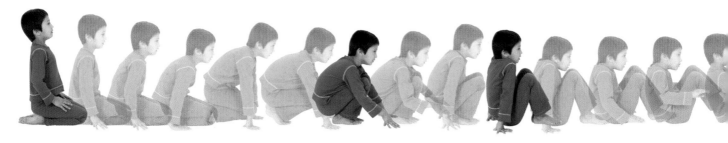

● Start from the resting kneeling position. Lift your chest, look straight ahead, and place your hands on your thighs. Take one full breath in and out.

● Lean forward and place your hands beside your knees, palms face down. Slowly lift your hips up and tuck your toes under. Shift your weight back into your heels so you are now in a squatting position.

● Begin to lower your hips down so that you move into a seated position. Keep your hands beside you for balance and support.

● Continue to look straight ahead, and keep your face relaxed. Now gently lift your feet off the floor so you are balancing on your pelvis.

■ ▶ **inhale** ▶ **exhale** ▶ **inhale** ▶

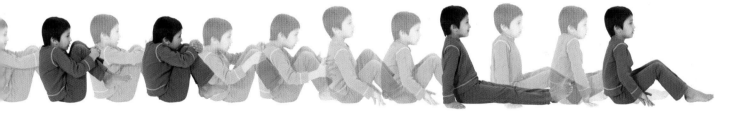

● At the same time, pick up your hands and wrap your arms around your legs. Hug them tight into your body as if you are squeezing out all your breath.

● Slowly release your hands like a flower bud opening its petals. Start to straighten your legs out.

● As you breathe out, straighten your legs fully so they are lying flat on the floor in front of you. This posture is traditionally called Dandasana, which means Seated Staff Pose.

● Place your hands beside your hips as you lift your chest. Start to bend your knees again as you begin to prepare for Boat Across Water.

▶ **exhale**   **inhale**   ▶   **exhale**   ▶   **inhale**

boat across water

This posture stretches the whole of the back of the body, in particular the muscles in your lower back. It also tones your belly. In order to protect your spine, it is very important to draw your abdomen in toward the spine. Lift your chest as high as you can so your back is straight.

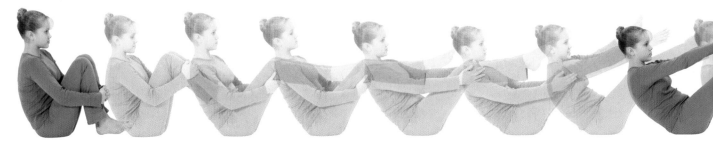

● Start in Flower Bud Closing. Your knees are bent and legs tucked in tight to your chest so your thighs are massaging your tummy. Keep your chest lifted and your face and shoulders relaxed.

● Tighten your tummy muscles as you begin to release your hands from around your legs. Lift your heels up so your shins are parallel to the floor as you begin to uncurl.

● Now straighten your arms so they are parallel to the floor. Draw your shoulders back and lift your chest as high as you can. Balance carefully as you start to straighten out your legs.

● Stretch your arms and legs out as straight as possible, aiming to create a V-shape with your body. Stretch out your hands as if they were oars for your boat. Take a full breath in the boat.

■   ▶   **begin to exhale**   ▶   **exhale and inhale**   ▶

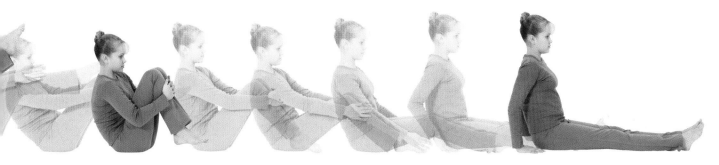

● Begin to bend the knees again so you can relax your back. Give yourself a tight hug as you return to the Flower Bud Closing position. This will relax your lower back.

● Keep looking straight ahead as you start slowly to release your clasp from around your shins.

● Gently start to straighten out your legs. Lift your chest up so your spine is as straight as possible and bring your hands down alongside your hips.

● Draw your shoulders back and straighten your arms. Flex your feet and press your knees into the ground. You are again in the classical Hatha yoga position Dandasana.

exhale ▶ **inhale** ▶ **exhale** ◼

bow and arrow

From Dandasana, the body is transformed to look like a bow and arrow. You hook the big toe and bend the knee, just as if you were drawing back a bow, ready to shoot an arrow. This movement is good for stretching the hips and lower back.

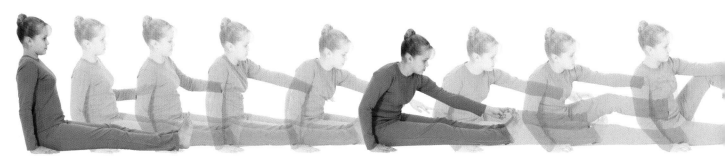

● Sharing the weight equally through the bones of each buttock, sit comfortably and steadily in Dandasana. Look straight ahead and lift your chest as you take a deep breath in.

● As you breathe out, reach for your left big toe. Use the first two fingers of your left hand to hook it (if you can't reach your big toe, then bend your knee so you can). Keep your right hand on the floor by your side.

● Keep your shoulders as relaxed as possible and get ready to bend your left knee and lift your left foot up off the floor.

● Lift your leg up as you start to transform your body to take on the shape of a bow and arrow.

■   **exhale** ▶ **begin to inhale** ▶ **inhale** ▶

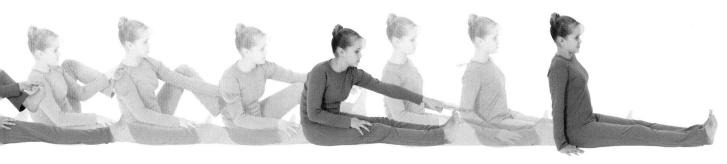

● As you breathe out, draw your left knee back as far as possible to give yourself a dip stretch in the hip. Keep your chest lifted all the while. Rest your right hand upon your right thigh.

● Keeping your eyes focussed on a still point in front of you, gradually bring your left leg back down in line with your right. As you do this, try to avoid hunching your back.

● Now, let go of your toe and draw your spine straight so it is vertical to the floor. Keep looking directly in front of you.

● Place your hands on the floor by your sides as you return to Dandasana. Relax your shoulders and take a deep breath in and out as you prepare to repeat the sequence on your right side.

exhale   ▶   **inhale**   ▶   **exhale**   ▶   **inhale and exhale**   ■

snap dragon closing

This safe forward bend resembles a flower nodding its head. Practicing it with the knees bent makes it very safe for your lower back. The posture releases and stretches your lower back and helps you to develop good alignment. As with all the postures, breathe freely and move smoothly, just like a flower swaying in the breeze.

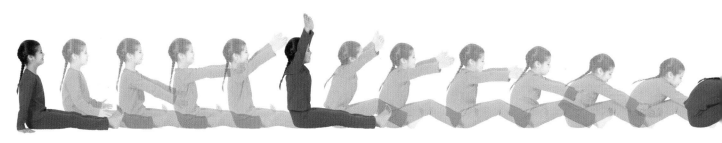

● Begin by sitting with your spine straight, like a plant stem. Stretch your legs out in front of you. Flex your feet by pushing your heels away from you. Spread your toes out like a fan.

● As you breathe in, slowly raise your arms forward, then up alongside your ears. As you reach your fingertips to the sky, stretch through the sides of your waist.

● As you gently lower your arms out in front of you, lean your chest forward. Keep your hips planted firmly on the ground and bend your knees slightly.

● With your knees slightly bent and your heels on the floor, gently rest your tummy on your thighs. Lower your straight arms onto your legs and clasp ankles. Without straining, drop your forehead onto your knees.

■　　▶　　　　**inhale**　　　　▶　　**exhale**　　　　▶

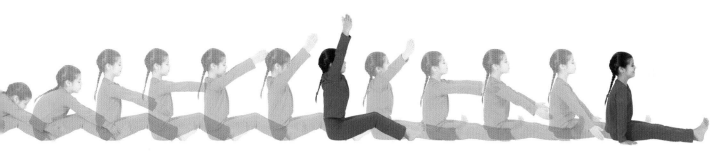

● Begin to lift your face up from your knees as you guide your upper body back up to a seated position. Keep your knees bent as you straighten out your spine and lift your arms.

● Now stretch your arms right up above your head as you take your in-breath deep into your chest.

● As you start to breathe out, lower your arms down again, in a slow and controlled way. At the same time, begin to straighten your legs.

● Place your hands alongside your hips, with your palms planted firmly into the ground. Lift your chest up and draw your shoulders back as if you were smiling from armpit to armpit.

inhale ▶ ▶ **exhale** ▶ ∎

spiralling seashells

This posture gives the body a great twist, just like a corkscrew. Its movement echoes the pattern of a spiralling seashell. The whole spine is massaged from bottom to top, which brings freedom and ease of movement. Twists help us to tune into the spine, the backbone of the body. Aim to move your body with awareness, smoothly and gracefully.

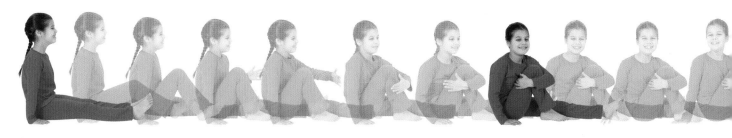

● Take a deep breath in and out to prepare. Relax your face and smile gently. Lengthen your neck, draw your shoulders back, and press your palms firmly into the ground.

● Begin to bend your right knee, bringing the right heel close into your hip. Your right knee is pointing up. Lift your left hand off the floor.

● Place your right hand on the floor just beneath you and hug your raised right leg with your left arm. Start to turn your chest to the right as you begin the twist.

● Squeeze your right thigh into your tummy to give it a good massage. Turn the fingers of your right hand away from your body so you can open your right shoulder.

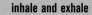 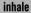 **inhale and exhale**   **inhale**   **exhale**

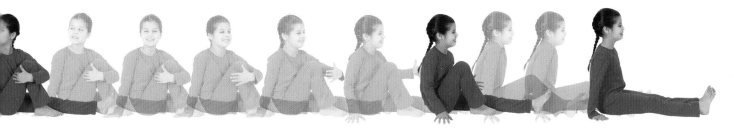

● Broaden both collarbones as you try to keep both shoulders level. Fill your lungs with fresh breath. As you breathe out, turn your chin over your right shoulder gently to exercise your neck muscles.

● As you continue breathing out, undo your twist. Move your head to look over your left shoulder. Release your left hand from your right leg.

● Bring your left hand back alongside your left hip. Face forward and start to straighten out your right leg

● Keep your face relaxed as you look straight ahead. Back in Dandasana, take a deep breath in and out, and then repeat the twist with your left leg.

inhale and exhale   ▶   ▶   ▶   **inhale and exhale**   ◼

frog sitting on rock

This posture stretches the spine forward and backward for strength and flexibility. By raising your hips, your body weight is carefully tipped upward and you roll onto the crown of your head. This movement flushes blood through the upper body, chest, neck, and head, while bringing flexibility to the shoulders. The movement finishes in a Seated Frog position, resting as if sitting on a lillypad.

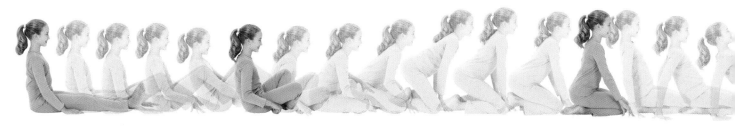

● Begin in Dandasana. Lift your chest, draw your shoulders back, stretch out your legs, and flex your feet.

● Cross your legs, tucking your heels into your hips. Begin to lean forward so you can place your hands on the floor beside your knees.

● Lean forward to lift your hips up off the floor. Undo your crossed legs so you can move into a kneeling position. Rest your hands on your thighs.

● Bring your hands back and place them just behind your hips. Plant them firmly into the floor for support. Begin to lean back to stretch open the abdomen. Lift your chest and let your head drop back behind you.

inhale　　　　　　　　　**exhale**

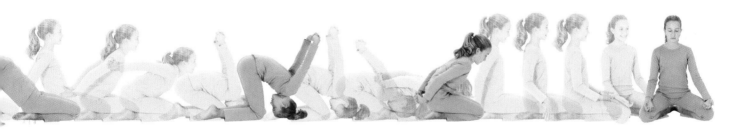

● Bring your chin back onto your chest. Ease your weight out of your hands again as you lean up to a kneeling position. At the peak of your in-breath, clasp your hands together behind you, interlocking your fingers.

● Fold your upper body over your thighs and lower your forehead onto the floor. Breathe in, lifting your hips to move into a Raised Child's Pose. Roll your body weight onto the crown of your head and raise your arms high.

● Having stretched your shoulders deeply and brought fresh blood to your brain, release your hands and come up into a seated position. Your hips are on your heels and your arms are resting by your side.

● Keep your spine straight as you separate your knees to sit like a frog on a rock. Place your hands on your thighs. Now, take a deep breath in and out, and smile peacefully.

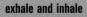 **inhale** ▶  **exhale and inhale** ▶ **exhale and inhale** ▶ **exhale**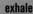

angels on your pillow

Yoga Nidra means dreamless sleep and this is what we are closing with in our final posture. We send you Angels on Your Pillow so that when you spring back to normal waking life, you are able to bring with you positivity and good energy.

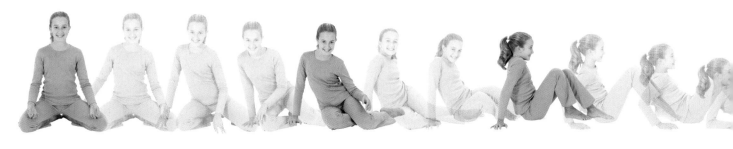

● Begin by sitting in Frog on Rock pose. Your knees are wide apart, your hands are on your thighs, your spine is tall and straight, and you are looking straight ahead of you.

● Ease out of your kneeling position by shifting your torso to your right as you drop your right thigh onto the floor. Rest your right hand on the floor beside you for support.

● Now raise your knees up off the floor. Keep them tucked up as you bring them to face toward you. Relax your belly and place your left hand beside your left hip.

● Begin to uncurl your spine like a fern into the mat. Bring your body down onto your elbows, but keep your chin tucked into your chest.

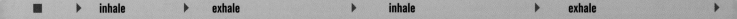

■ ▶ **inhale** ▶ **exhale** ▶ **inhale** ▶ **exhale** ▶

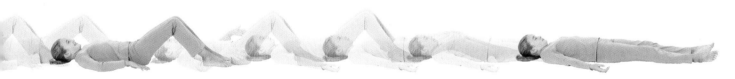

● Straighten your arms beside you without any jerky or forced movements. Relax your shoulder bones down into the floor like stones. Uncurl your neck so the back of the head rests comfortably on the floor.

● Look straight up so your neck is in line with your spine. Ease your shoulders away from your ears. Relax the whole of your back deep into the floor. Your arms are by your side, palms face upward.

● Having relaxed your spine, start to straighten out your legs. Slide your heels away from you so your feet are hip-width apart. Relax your hips and let the bones of your legs become heavy as they sink deeper into the floor.

● With arms and legs fully relaxed, let your feet fall gently outward. Take a deep breath in and out. Imagine you are floating on water as you surrender your limbs into the floor, resting as if you have angels on your pillow.

inhale ▶ **exhale** ▶ **inhale and exhale** ■

index

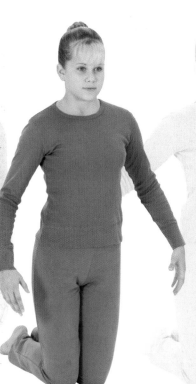

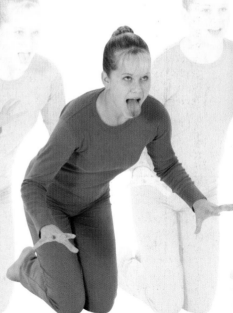